Keto Vegetarian Diet for Beginners

Lose Weight Naturally with Delicious Low-Carb Recipes

Lauren Bellisario

Table of Contents

Blueberry Chia Pudding

Preparation time: 3 minutes + 4 hours refrigeration

Servings: 2

Nutritional Values (Per Serving):

- Calories:64
- Total Fat:7.3 g
- Saturated Fat: 5.3g
- Total Carbs:3 g
- Dietary Fiber: 2g
- Sugar: 2g
- Protein: 3g
- Sodium: 300mg

Ingredients:

- ¾ cup coconut milk
- ½ tsp vanilla extract
- ½ cup blueberries
- 2 tbsp chia seeds
- Chopped walnuts to garnish

Directions:

1. Mix all the Ingredients in a medium bowl except for the walnuts.
2. Share the mixture into two breakfast jars, cover, and refrigerate for 4 hours or until the pudding gels.
3. Remove when ready to enjoy, top with some blueberries, walnuts, and serve immediately.

Bulletproof Coffee

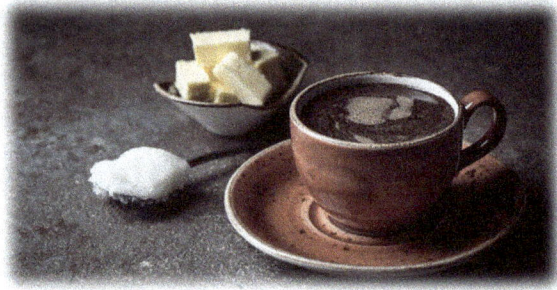

Preparation time: 3 minutes

Serving: 2

Nutritional Values (Per Serving):

- Calories: 307
- Total Fat:29.9 g
- Saturated Fat:11.3 g
- Total Carbs: 9 g
- Dietary Fiber: 3g
- Sugar: 4g
- Protein:6 g
- Sodium: 8mg

Ingredients:

- 2 ½ heaping tbsp. ground bulletproof coffee beans
- 1 cup water
- 1 tbsp MCT oil

- 2 tbsp unsalted butter

Directions:

1. Using a coffee maker, brew one cup of coffee with the ground coffee beans and water.
2. Transfer the coffee to a blender and add the MCT oil and butter. Blend the mixture until frothy and smooth.
3. Divide the drink into two teacups and enjoy immediately.

Eggplant Pomodoro

Preparation time: 5 min

Cooking time: 15 min

Serves: 4

Nutritional Values (Per Serving):

- Kcal: 101
- Fat: 7 g.
- Protein: 1 g.
- Carbs: 9 g.

Ingredients:

- 1 Medium Eggplant, diced
- 1 cup Diced Tomatoes
- ½ cup Black Olives, sliced
- 4 cloves Garlic, minced
- 2 tbsp Red Wine Vinegar

- pinch of Red Pepper Flakes
- Salt and Pepper to taste
- 2 tbsp Olive Oil
- 4 cups Shirataki Pasta
- Fresh Parsley for garnish

Directions:

1. Heat olive oil in a pan.
2. Sautee garlic and red pepper flakes until aromatic.
3. Add eggplants, tomatoes, olives and red wine vinegar. Stir until eggplants are soft.
4. Toss shirataki into the pan.
5. Season with salt and pepper.
6. Garnish with chopped fresh parsley for serving.

Vegetable Char Siu

Preparation time: 5 min

Cooking time: 15 min

Serves: 4

Nutritional Values (Per Serving):

- Kcal: 100
- Fat: 7 g.
- Protein: 1 g.
- Carbs: 9 g.

Ingredients:

- 100 grams Raw Jackfruit, deseeded and rinsed
- 100 grams Cucumbers, cut into thin strips
- 50 grams Red Bell Pepper, cut into thin strips
- 2 cloves Garlic, minced
- 1 Shallot, minced
- ¼ cup Char Siu Sauce
- ¼ cup Water
- 2 tbsp Peanut Oil

Directions:

1. Heat peanut oil in a pan.
2. Add jackfruit and stir until slightly brown.
3. Add garlic and shallots and sautee until aromatic.
4. Add water and char siu sauce. Simmer until jackfruit is tender.
5. Shred jackfruit with forks.
6. Toss in cucumbers and bell peppers.

Soy Sauce Tofu

Preparation time: 5 min

Cooking time: 15 min

Serves: 6

Nutritional Values (Per Serving):

- Kcal: 249
- Fat: 18 g.
- Protein: 14 g.
- Carbs: 9 g.

Ingredients:

- 500 grams Firm Tofu, pressed and drained
- ¼ cup Soy Sauce
- ¼ cup Red Wine Vinegar
- ¼ cup Tomato Paste
- 1 tsp Paprika
- 1 tsp Chili Powder 1 tsp Garlic Powder
- ½ tsp Onion Powder 1 tsp Cumin Powder
- ½ tsp Black Pepper

- ½ tsp Salt
- ¼ cup Olive Oil

Directions:

1. Crumble tofu in a bowl. Mix in all ingredients except for the olive oil.
2. Heat olive oil in a non-stick pan.
3. Add tofu mix and stir for 10-15 minutes.
4. Serve in tacos, wraps, burritos, or rice bowls.

Vietnamese "Vermicelli" Salad

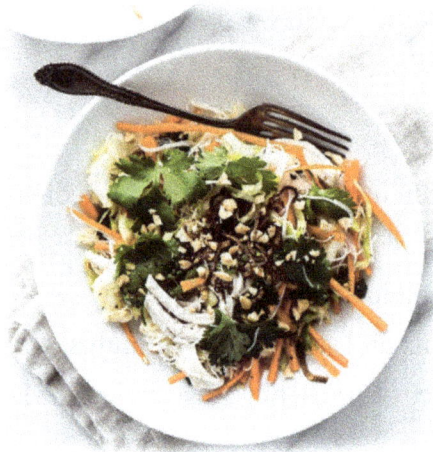

Preparation time: 5 min

Cooking time:

Serves: 4

Nutritional Values (Per Serving):

- Kcal: 249
- Fat: 11 g.
- Protein: 5 g.
- Carbs: 8 g.

Ingredients:

- 100 grams Carrot, sliced into thin strips
- 200 grams Cucumbers, spiralized
- 2 tbsp Roasted Peanuts, roughly chopped
- ¼ cup Fresh Mint, chopped
- ¼ cup Fresh Cilantro, chopped
- 1 tbsp Stevia
- 2 tbsp Fresh Lime Juice
- 1 tbsp Vegan Fish Sauce
- 2 cloves Garlic, minced
- 1 Green Chili, deseeded and minced
- 2 tbsp Sesame Oil

Directions:

1. Whisk together sugar, lime juice, sesame oil, fish sauce, minced garlic, and chopped chili. Set aside.
2. In a bowl, toss together cucumbers, carrots, cucumbers, peanuts, mint, cilantro, and prepared dressing.
3. Serve chilled.

Enoki Mushroom and Snow Pea Soba

Preparation time: 5 min

Cooking time: 5 min

Serves: 2

Nutritional Values (Per Serving):

- Kcal: 167
- Fat: 14 g.
- Protein: 4 g.
- Carbs: 8 g.

Ingredients:

- 75 grams Snow Peas
- 100 grams Shimeji Mushrooms
- 2 tsp Minced Ginger
- ¼ cup Mirin
- 3 tbsp Light Soy Sauce
- 1 tsp Erythritol

- 1 tbsp Sesame Oil
- 1 tbsp Vegetable Oil

Directions:

1. Heat vegetable oil in a wok. Sautee ginger until aromatic.
2. Add snow peas and stir fry for 1-2 minutes.
3. Add shimeji mushrooms and stir for another minute.
4. Add mirin, soy sauce, and erythritol.
5. Turn off the heat and drizzle in sesame oil.

Spicy Carrot Noodles

Preparation time: 20 minutes

Servings: 3

Nutritional Values (Per Serving):

- Calories 450
- Fat 45 g
- Carbohydrates 14 g
- Sugar 6 g
- Protein 2 g
- Cholesterol 0 mg

Ingredients:

- 5 medium carrots
- 4 tbsp red chili pepper flakes, crushed
- 2/3 cup olive oil
- 1/4 cup vinegar
- 3 garlic cloves, chopped
- 1/4 cup fresh spring onions, chopped

- 1/2 cup basil leaves
- 1 cup fresh parsley Salt

Directions:

1. Add red chili flakes, oil, vinegar, garlic, spring onions, basil, and parsley in a blender and blend until smooth. Pour paste into a large bowl.
2. Add water in a large saucepan with little salt and bring to boil.
3. Peel carrots and using spiralizer make noodles.
4. Add carrot noodles in boiling water and blanch for 2 minutes or until softened.
5. Add cooked noodles in large bowl and toss mix well with paste.
6. Serve immediately and enjoy.

Creamy Zucchini Quiche

Preparation time: 120 minutes

Servings: 8

Nutritional Values (Per Serving):

- Calories 253
- Fat 21 g
- Carbohydrates 6 g
- Sugar 3 g
- Protein 11 g
- Cholesterol 76 mg

Ingredients:

- 2 lbs zucchini, thinly sliced
- 1 1/2 cup almond milk
- 2 large eggs
- 2 cups cheddar cheese, shredded Pepper
- Salt

Directions:

1. Preheat the oven to 375 F.
2. Season zucchini with pepper and salt and set aside for 30 minutes.
3. In a large bowl, beat eggs with almond milk, pepper, and salt.
4. Add shredded cheddar cheese and stir well.
5. Spray quiche pan with cooking spray and arrange zucchini slices in quiche pan.
6. Pour egg and milk mixture over zucchini the sprinkle shredded cheese.
7. Bake in preheated oven for 60 minutes or until quiche is lightly golden brown.
8. Serve warm and enjoy.

Simple Garlic Cauliflower Couscous

Preparation time: 30 minutes

Servings: 3

Nutritional Values (Per Serving):

- Calories 51
- Fat 0.2 g
- Carbohydrates 10 g
- Sugar 4 g
- Protein 3 g
- Cholesterol 0 mg

Ingredients:

- 1 medium cauliflower head, cut into florets
- 2 tsp parsley, dried
- 2 tsp garlic, dried
- Salt

Directions:

1. Add cauliflower florets into the food processor and process until it looks like couscous.
2. Heat large pan over medium-low heat.
3. Add cauliflower couscous, parsley, and garlic in the pan and cook until softened.
4. Stir well and season with salt.
5. Serve and enjoy.

Brussels Sprouts

Preparation time: 10 minutes

Cooking time: 3 hours

Servings: 12

Nutritional Values (Per Serving):

- Calories 100
- Fat 4
- Fiber 4
- Carbs 14
- Protein 3

Ingredients:

- 1 cup red onion, chopped
- 2 pounds Brussels sprouts, trimmed and halved
- A pinch of salt and black pepper
- ¼ cup apple juice

- 3 tablespoons olive oil
- ¼ cup maple syrup
- 1 tablespoon thyme, chopped

Directions:

1. In your slow cooker, mix Brussels sprouts with onion, salt, pepper and apple juice, toss, cover and cook on Low for 3 hours.
2. In a bowl, mix maple syrup with oil and thyme, whisk really well and add over Brussels sprouts.
3. Toss well, divide between plates and serve as a side dish.
4. Enjoy!

Beets and Carrots

Preparation time: 10 minutes

Cooking time: 7 hours

Servings: 8

Nutritional Values (Per Serving):

- Calories 125
- Fat 0
- Fiber 4
- Carbs 28
- Protein 3

Ingredients:

- 2 tablespoons stevia
- ¾ cup pomegranate juice
- 2 teaspoons ginger, grated
- 2 and ½ pounds beets, peeled and cut into wedges
- 12 ounces carrots, cut into medium wedges

Directions:

1. In your slow cooker, mix beets with carrots, ginger, stevia and pomegranate juice, toss, cover and cook on Low for 7 hours.
2. Divide between plates and serve as a side dish.
3. Enjoy!

Italian Veggie Side Dish

Preparation time: 10 minutes

Cooking time: 6 hours

Servings: 8

Nutritional Values (Per Serving):

- Calories 364
- Fat 12
- Fiber 10
- Carbs 45
- Protein 21

Ingredients:

- 38 ounces canned cannellini beans, drained
- 1 yellow onion, chopped
- ¼ cup basil pesto
- 19 ounces canned fava beans, drained
- 4 garlic cloves, minced
- 1 and ½ teaspoon Italian seasoning, dried and crushed
- 1 tomato, chopped

- 15 ounces already cooked polenta, cut into medium pieces
- 2 cups spinach
- 1 cup radicchio, torn

Directions:

1. In your slow cooker, mix cannellini beans with fava beans, basil pesto, onion, garlic, Italian seasoning, polenta, tomato, spinach and radicchio, toss, cover and cook on Low for 6 hours.
2. Divide between plates and serve as a side dish.
3. Enjoy!

Acorn Squash and Great Sauce

Preparation time: 10 minutes

Cooking time: 6 hours

Servings: 4

Nutritional Values (Per Serving):

- Calories 325
- Fat 6
- Fiber 3
- Carbs 28
- Protein 3

Ingredients:

- 2 acorn squash, halved, deseeded and cut into medium wedges
- ¼ cup raisins
- 16 ounces cranberry sauce
- ¼ cup orange marmalade
- A pinch of salt and black pepper
- ¼ teaspoon cinnamon powder

Directions:

1. In your slow cooker, mix squash with raisins, cranberry sauce, orange marmalade, salt, pepper and cinnamon powder, toss, cover and cook on Low for 6 hours.
2. Stir again, divide between plates and serve as a side dish.
3. Enjoy!

Red Beans Rice

Preparation time: 10 minutes

Cooking time: 7 hours

Servings: 12

Nutritional Values (Per Serving):

- Calories 168
- Fat 5
- Fiber 4
- Carbs 25
- Protein 6

Ingredients:

- ½ cup wild rice
- ½ cup barley
- 2/3 cup wheat berries
- 27 ounces veggie stock
- 2 cups baby lima beans
- 1 red bell pepper, chopped
- 1 yellow onion, chopped

- 1 tablespoon olive oil
- A pinch of salt and black pepper
- 1 teaspoon sage, dried and crushed
- 4 garlic cloves, minced

Directions:

1. In your slow cooker, mix rice with barley, wheat berries, lima beans, bell pepper, onion, oil, salt, pepper, sage and garlic, stir, cover and cook on Low for 7 hours.
2. Stir one more time, divide between plates and serve as a side dish.
3. Enjoy!

Special Potatoes Mix

Preparation time: 10 minutes

Cooking time: 7 hours

Servings: 10

Nutritional Values (Per Serving):

- Calories 351
- Fat 8
- Fiber 5
- Carbs 48
- Protein 2

Ingredients:

- 2 green apples, cored and cut into wedges
- 3 pounds sweet potatoes, peeled and cut into medium wedges
- 1 cup coconut cream
- ½ cup dried cherries
- 1 cup apple butter
- 1 and ½ teaspoon pumpkin pie spice

Directions:

1. In your slow cooker, mix sweet potatoes with green apples, cream, cherries, apple butter and spice, toss, cover and cook on Low for 7 hours.
2. Toss, divide between plates and serve as a side dish.
3. Enjoy!

Creamy Corn

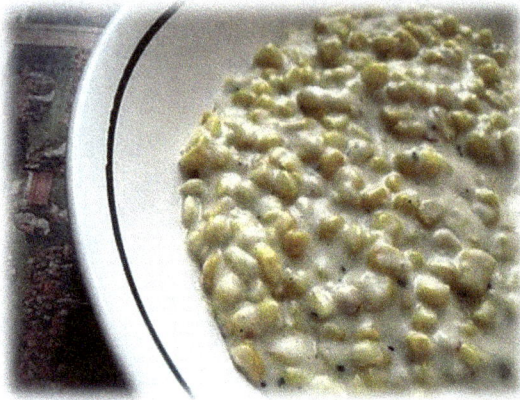

Preparation time: 10 minutes

Cooking time: 3 hours

Servings: 6

Nutritional Values (Per Serving):

- Calories 200
- Fat 5
- Fiber 7
- Carbs 12
- Protein 4

Ingredients:

- 50 ounces corn
- 1 cup almond milk
- 1 tablespoon stevia
- 8 ounces coconut cream
- A pinch of white pepper

Directions:

1. In your slow cooker, mix corn with almond milk, stevia, cream and white pepper, toss, cover and cook on High for 3 hours.
2. Divide between plates and serve as a side dish.
3. Enjoy!

Broccoli Stew

Preparation time: 10 minutes

Cooking time: 40 minutes

Servings: 4

Nutritional Values (Per Serving):

- Calories – 150
- Fat – 4
- Fiber – 2
- Carbs – 5
- Protein - 12

Ingredients:

- 1 broccoli head, separated into florets
- 2 teaspoons coriander seeds
- A drizzle of olive oil
- 1 onion, peeled and chopped

- Salt and ground black pepper, to taste
- A pinch of red pepper, crushed
- 1 small ginger piece, peeled, and chopped
- 1 garlic clove, peeled and minced
- 28 ounces canned pureed tomatoes

Directions:

1. Put water in a pot, add the salt, bring to a boil over medium-high heat, add the broccoli florets, steam them for 2 minutes, transfer them to a bowl filled with ice water, drain them, and leave aside.
2. Heat up a pan over medium-high heat, add the coriander seeds, toast them for 4 minutes, transfer to a grinder, ground them, and set aside as well.
3. Heat up a pot with the oil over medium heat, add the onions, salt, pepper, and red pepper, stir, and cook for 7 minutes.
4. Add the ginger, garlic, and coriander seeds, stir, and cook for 3 minutes.
5. Add the tomatoes, bring to a boil, and simmer for 10 minutes.
6. Add the broccoli, stir and cook the stew for 12 minutes.
7. Divide into bowls and serve.

Bok Choy Soup

Preparation time: 10 minutes

Cooking time: 15 minutes

Servings: 4

Nutritional Values (Per Serving):

- Calories – 100
- Fat – 3
- Fiber – 1
- Carbs – 2
- Protein - 6

Ingredients:

- 3 cups beef stock
- 1 onion, peeled and chopped
- 1 bunch bok choy, chopped
- 1½ cups mushrooms, chopped
- Salt and ground black pepper, to taste
- ½ tablespoon red pepper flakes
- 3 tablespoons coconut aminos

- 3 tablespoons Parmesan cheese, grated
- 2 tablespoons Worcestershire sauce
- 2 bacon strips, chopped

Directions:

1. Heat up a pot over medium-high heat, add the bacon, stir, cook until it until crispy, transfer to paper towels, and drain the grease.
2. Heat up the pot again over medium heat, add the mushrooms and onions, stir, and cook for 5 minutes.
3. Add the stock, bok choy, coconut aminos, salt, pepper, pepper flakes, and Worcestershire sauce, stir, cover, and cook until bok choy is tender.
4. Ladle the soup into bowls, sprinkle Parmesan cheese, and bacon, and serve.

Bok Choy Stir-fry

Preparation time: 10 minutes

Cooking time: 7 minutes

Servings: 2

Nutritional Values (Per Serving):

- Calories – 50
- Fat – 1
- Fiber – 1
- Carbs – 2
- Protein - 2

Ingredients:

- 2 garlic cloves, peeled and minced
- 2 cup bok choy, chopped
- 2 bacon slices, chopped
- Salt and ground black pepper, to taste
- A drizzle of avocado oil

Directions:

1. Heat up a pan with the oil over medium heat, add the bacon, stir, and brown until crispy, transfer to paper towels, and drain the grease.
2. Return the pan to medium heat, add the garlic and bok choy, stir, and cook for 4 minutes.
3. Add the salt, pepper, and return the bacon to the pan, stir, cook for 1 minute, divide on plates, and serve.

Cream of Celery Soup

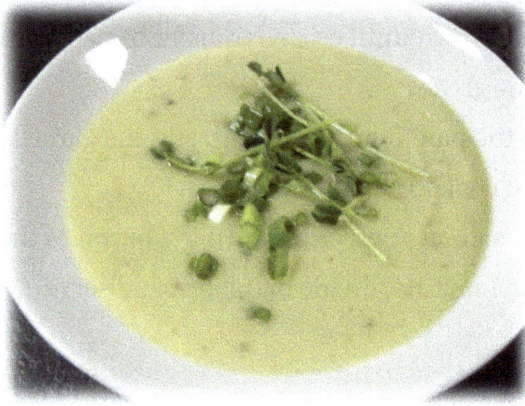

Preparation time: 10 minutes

Cooking time: 40 minutes

Servings: 4

Nutritional Values (Per Serving):

- Calories – 150
- Fat – 3
- Fiber – 1
- Carbs – 2
- Protein - 6

Ingredients:

- 1 bunch celery, chopped
- Salt and ground black pepper, to taste
- 3 bay leaves
- ½ garlic head, peeled, and chopped
- 2 onions, peeled and chopped
- 4 cups chicken stock
- ¾ cup heavy cream
- 2 tablespoons butter

Directions:

1. Heat up a pot with the butter over medium-high heat, add the onions, salt, and pepper, stir, and cook for 5 minutes.
2. Add the bay leaves, garlic, and celery, stir, and cook for 15 minutes.
3. Add the stock, more salt and pepper, stir, cover the pot, reduce the heat, and simmer for 20 minutes.
4. Add the cream, stir, and blend everything using an immersion blender.
5. Ladle into soup bowls and serve.

Celery Stew

Preparation time: 10 minutes

Cooking time: 30 minutes

Servings: 6

Nutritional Values (Per Serving):

- Calories – 170
- Fat – 7
- Fiber – 4
- Carbs – 6
- Protein - 10

Ingredients:

- 1 celery bunch, chopped
- 1 onion, peeled and chopped
- 1 bunch green onion, peeled and chopped
- 4 garlic cloves, peeled and minced
- Salt and ground black pepper, to taste
- 1 fresh parsley bunch, chopped
- 2 fresh mint bunches, chopped

- 3 dried Persian lemons, pricked with a fork
- 2 cups water
- 2 teaspoons chicken bouillon
- 4 tablespoons olive oil

Directions:

1. Heat up a pot with the oil over medium-high heat, add the onion, green onions, and garlic, stir, and cook for 6 minutes.
2. Add the celery, Persian lemons, chicken bouillon, salt, pepper, and water, stir, cover pot, and simmer on medium heat for 20 minutes.
3. Add the parsley and mint, stir, and cook for 10 minutes.
4. Divide into bowls and serve.

Black Bean Soup with a Splash

Preparation time: 5 Minutes

Cooking time: 45 Minutes

Servings: 4 To 6

Ingredients:

- 1 tablespoon olive oil
- 1 medium onion, finely chopped
- 1 celery rib, finely chopped
- 2 medium carrots, finely chopped
- 1 small green bell pepper, finely chopped
- 2 garlic cloves, minced
- 1 teaspoon dried thyme
- 1 teaspoon salt
- 1/4 teaspoon ground cayenne
- 2 tablespoons minced fresh parsley, for garnish
- 1/3 cup dry sherry

- 4 cups vegetable broth (homemade, store-bought, or water)
- 4½ cups cooked or 3 (15.5-ounce) cans black beans, drained and rinsed

Directions:

1. In a large soup pot, heat the oil over medium heat. Add the onion, celery, carrots, bell pepper, and garlic. Cover and cook until tender, stirring occasionally, about 10 minutes. Add the broth, beans, thyme, salt, and cayenne. Bring to a boil, then reduce the heat to low and simmer, uncovered, until the soup has thickened, about 45 minutes.
2. Puree the soup in the pot with an immersion blender or in a blender or food processor, in batches if necessary, and return to the pot. Reheat if necessary.
3. Ladle the soup into bowls and garnish with parsley. Serve accompanied by the sherry.

Cream of Tomato Soup

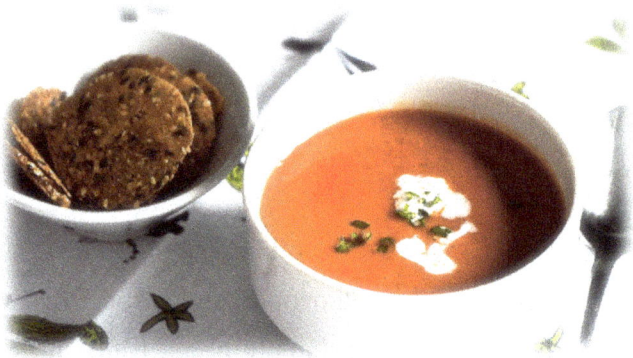

Preparation time: 5 Minutes

Cooking time: 5 Minutes

Servings: 2

Nutrition per Serving (2 cups):

- Calories: 90
- Protein: 4g
- Total fat: 3g
- Saturated fat: 0g
- Carbohydrates: 16g
- Fiber: 4g

Ingredients:

- 1 (28-ounce) can crushed, diced, or whole peeled tomatoes, undrained
- 1 to 2 teaspoons dried herbs
- 2 to 3 teaspoons onion powder (optional)
- ¾ to 1 cup unsweetened nondairy milk
- ½ teaspoon salt, or to taste
- Freshly ground black pepper

Directions:

1. Preparing the ingredients.
2. Pour the tomatoes and their juices into a large pot and bring them to near-boiling over medium heat.
3. Add the dried herbs, onion powder (if using), milk, salt, and pepper to taste. Stir to combine. If you used diced or whole tomatoes, use a hand blender to purée the soup until smooth. (Alternatively, let the soup cool for a few minutes, then transfer to a countertop blender.) Leftovers will keep in an airtight container for up to 1 week in the refrigerator or up to 1 month in the freezer (though if you want leftovers for this soup, you might want to double the recipe).

Southern Succotash Stew

Preparation time: 5 Minutes

Cooking time: 60 Minutes

Servings: 4

Ingredients:

- 8 ounces tempeh
- 2 tablespoons olive oil
- 1 large sweet yellow onion, finely chopped
- 2 medium russet potatoes, peeled and cut into 1/2-inch dice
- 2 carrots, cut into 1/4-inch slices
- 1 (14.5-ounce) can diced tomatoes, drained
- 1 (16-ounce) package frozen succotash
- 2 cups vegetable broth or water
- 2 tablespoons soy sauce
- 1 teaspoon dry mustard
- 1/2 teaspoon dried thyme
- 1/2 teaspoon ground allspice
- 1/4 teaspoon ground cayenne
- Salt and freshly ground black pepper
- 1/2 teaspoon liquid smoke

Directions:

1. In a medium saucepan of simmering water, cook the empeh for 30 minutes. Drain, pat dry, and cut into 1-inch dice.

2. In a large skillet, heat 1 tablespoon of the oil over medium heat. Add the tempeh and cook until browned on both sides, about 10 minutes. Set aside.

3. In a large saucepan, heat the remaining 1 tablespoon oil over medium heat. Add the onion and cook until softened, 5 minutes. Add the potatoes, carrots, tomatoes, succotash, broth, soy sauce, mustard, sugar, thyme, allspice, and cayenne. Season with salt and pepper to taste. Bring to a boil, then reduce heat to low and add the tempeh. Simmer, covered, until the vegetables are tender, stirring occasionally, about 45 minutes.

4. About 10 minutes before the stew is finished cooking, stir in the liquid smoke. Taste, adjusting seasonings if necessary. Serve immediately.

Seitan keto

Preparation time: 25 minutes + overtime chilling time **Serving size:** 4

Nutritional Values (Per Serving):

- Calories:273
- Total Fat:20g
- Saturated Fat:11.6g
- Total Carbs:6g
- Dietary Fiber:1g
- Sugar:4g
- Protein:17g
- Sodium:931mg

Ingredients:

For the keto pasta:

- 1 cup shredded mozzarella cheese
- 1 egg yolk

For the seitan and vegetables:

- 1 tbsp sesame oil
- 3 seitan, cut into ¼-inch strips
- Salt and black pepper to taste
- 1 red bell pepper, deseeded and thinly sliced
- 1 yellow bell pepper, deseeded and thinly sliced
- 1 cup green beans, trimmed and halved
- 1 garlic clove, minced
- 1-inch ginger knob, peeled and grated
- 4 green onions, chopped
- 1 tsp toasted sesame seeds to garnish

For the sauce:

- 3 tbsp coconut aminos
- 2 tsp sesame oil
- 2 tsp sugar-free maple syrup
- 1 tsp fresh ginger paste

Directions:

For the pasta:

1. Pour the cheese into a medium safe-microwave bowl and melt in the microwave for 35 minutes or until melted.

2. Take out the bowl and allow cooling for 1 minute only to warm the cheese but not cool completely. Mix in the egg yolk until well-combined.

3. Lay a parchment paper on a flat surface, pour the cheese mixture on top and cover with another parchment paper. Using a rolling pin, flatten the dough into 1/8-inch thickness.

4. Take off the parchment paper and cut the dough into thin spaghetti strands. Place in a bowl and refrigerate overnight.

5. When ready to cook, bring 2 cups of water to a boil in medium saucepan and add the pasta. Cook for 40 seconds to 1 minute and then drain through a colander. Run cold water over the pasta and set aside to cool.

For the seitan and vegetables:

6. Heat the sesame oil in a large skillet, season the seitan with salt, black pepper, and sear in the oil on both sides until brown, 5 minutes. Transfer to a plate and set aside.

7. Mix in the bell peppers, green beans and cook until sweaty, 3 minutes. Stir in the garlic, ginger, green onions and cook until fragrant, 1 minute.

8. Add the seitan and pasta to the skillet and toss well.

9. In a small bowl, toss the sauce's **Ingredients:** the coconut aminos, sesame oil, maple syrup, and ginger paste.

10. Pour the mixture over the seitan mixture and toss well; cook for 1 minute.

11. Dish the food onto serving plates and garnish with the sesame seeds. Serve warm.

Pasta & Cheese Mushroom

Preparation time: 1 hour 45 minutes + overtime chilling **Serving size:** 4

Nutritional Values (Per Serving):

- Calories:647
- Total Fat:56.5g
- Saturated Fat:32g
- Total Carbs:6g
- Dietary Fiber:1g
- Sugar:2g
- Protein:30g
- Sodium:609mg

Ingredients:

For the keto macaroni:

- 1 cup shredded mozzarella cheese
- 1 egg yolk

For the pulled mushroom mac and cheese:

- 2 tbsp olive oil
- 1 lb mushroom
- Salt and black pepper to taste
- 1 tsp dried thyme
- 1 cup vegetable broth
- 2 tbsp butter
- 2 medium shallots, minced
- 2 garlic cloves, minced
- 1 cup water
- 1 cup grated cheddar cheese
- 4 oz dairy- free cream cheese, room temperature
- 1 cup coconut cream
- ½ tsp white pepper
- ½ tsp nutmeg powder
- 2 tbsp chopped parsley

Directions:

For the keto macaroni:

1. Pour the cheese into a medium safe-microwave bowl and melt in the microwave for 35 minutes or until melted.

2. Take out the bowl and allow cooling for 1 minute only to warm the cheese but not cool completely. Mix in the egg yolk until well-combined.

3. Lay a parchment paper on a flat surface, pour the cheese mixture on top and cover with another parchment paper. Using a rolling pin, flatten the dough into 1/8-inch thickness.

4. Take off the parchment paper and cut the dough into small cubes of the size of macaroni. Place in a bowl and refrigerate overnight.

5. When ready to cook, bring 2 cups of water to a boil in medium saucepan and add the keto macaroni. Cook for 40 seconds to 1 minute and then drain through a colander. Run cold water over the pasta and set aside to cool.

For the mushroom mac and cheese:

6. Heat the olive oil in a large pot, season the mushroom with salt, black pepper, thyme, and sear in the oil on both sides until brown. Pour on the vegetable broth, cover, and cook over low heat for 15 minutes or until softened. When ready, remove the mushroom onto a plate and set aside.

7. Preheat the oven to 380 F.

8. Melt the butter in a large skillet and sauté the shallots until softened. Stir in the garlic and cook until fragrant, 30 seconds.

9. Pour in the water to deglaze the pot and then stir in half of the cheddar cheese and dairy- free cream cheese until melted,

4 minutes. Mix in the coconut cream and season with salt, black pepper, white pepper, and nutmeg powder.

10. Add the pasta, mushroom, and half of the parsley to the mixture; combine well.

11. Pour the mixture into a baking dish and cover the top with the remaining cheddar cheese. Bake in the oven until the cheese melts and the food bubbly, 15 to 20 minutes.

12. Remove from the oven, allow cooling for 2 minutes and garnish with the

13. parsley.

14. Serve warm.

Cranberry-Carrot Salad

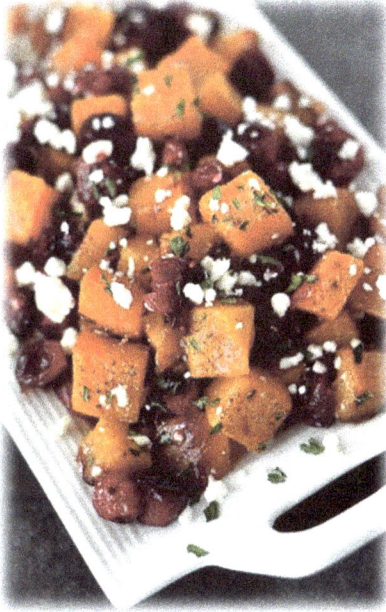

Preparation time: 15 Minutes

Cooking time: 0 Minutes

Servings: 4

Ingredients:

- 1 pound carrots, shredded
- 1 cup sweetened dried cranberries
- 1/2 cup toasted walnut pieces
- 2 tablespoons fresh lemon juice
- 3 tablespoons toasted walnut oil
- 1/8 teaspoon freshly ground black pepper

Directions:

1. In a large bowl, combine the carrots, cranberries, and walnuts. Set aside. In a small bowl, whisk together the lemon juice, walnut oil and pepper. Pour the dressing over the salad, toss gently to combine and serve.

Almond Crunch Chopped Kale Salad

Preparation time: 10 Minutes

Cooking time: 10 Minutes

Servings: 4

Ingredients:

For The Dressing

- ¼ cup tahini
- 2 tablespoons Dijon mustard 2 tablespoons maple syrup
- 1 tablespoon lemon juice
- ¼ teaspoon salt

For The Almond Crunch

- ½ cup finely chopped raw almonds
- 2 teaspoons soy sauce or gluten-free tamari 1 teaspoon maple syrup
- ¼ teaspoon sea salt

For The Salad

- 1 bunch lacinato kale, stemmed and roughly chopped 1 green apple, cored and thinly sliced

Directions:

1.   Preheat the oven to 325°F. Line a baking sheet with parchment paper.

For the the dressing:

2.   Whisk together all the dressing ingredients in a small bowl and set aside.

For the almond crunch:

3.   Mix together all the almond crunch ingredients in a medium bowl and spread out evenly on the prepared baking sheet. Bake for 5 to 7 minutes, until slightly darker in color and crunchy. Let cool for 3 minutes.

4.   To make the salad: In a large bowl, mix together the kale and apples. Toss with the dressing and top with the almond crunch.

Apple-Sunflower Spinach Salad

Preparation time: 5 Minutes

Cooking time: 0 Minutes

Servings: 1

Nutrition per Serving:

- Calories: 444
- Protein: 7g
- Total fat: 28g
- Saturated fat: 3g
- Carbohydrates: 53g
- Fiber: 8g

Ingredients:

- 1 cup baby spinach
- ½ apple, cored and chopped
- ¼ red onion, thinly sliced (optional)
- 2 tablespoons sunflower seeds or Cinnamon-Lime Sunflower Seeds

- 2 tablespoons dried cranberries
- 2 tablespoons Raspberry Vinaigrette

Directions:

1. Arrange the spinach on a plate. Top with the apple, red onion (if using), sunflower seeds, and cranberries, and drizzle with the vinaigrette.

Brussels sprouts Chips

Preparation time: 10 minutes

Cooking time: 10 minutes

Servings: 2

Nutritional Values (Per Serving):

- Calories: 101
- Fat: 7.3g
- Cabs: 8.6g
- Protein: 3.2g

Ingredients:

- 10 Brussels sprouts split leaves
- 1 tbsp. olive oil
- ¼ tsp. sea salt

Directions:

1. Preheat your oven to 350° Fahrenheit.
2. Toss Brussels sprouts with olive oil.
3. Season Brussels sprouts with salt. Spread Brussels sprouts in a baking dish and bake in preheated oven for 10 minutes.
4. Serve and enjoy!

Zaatar Popcorn

Preparation time: 10 minutes

Cooking time: 0 minute

Servings: 8

Nutritional Values (Per Serving):

- Calories:150 Cal
- Fat: 9 g
- Carbs: 15 g
- Protein: 2 g
- Fiber: 4 g

Ingredients:

- 8 cups popped popcorns
- 1/4 cup za'atar spice blend
- ¾ teaspoon salt
- 4 tablespoons olive oil

Directions:

1. Place all the ingredients except for popcorns in a large bowl and whisk until combined.
2. Then add popcorns, toss until well coated, and serve straight away.

Potato Chips

Preparation time: 10 minutes

Cooking time: 20 minutes

Servings: 2

Nutritional Values (Per Serving):

- Calories: 600 Cal
- Fat: 30 g
- Carbs: 78 g
- Protein: 9 g
- Fiber: 23 g

Ingredients:

- 3 medium potatoes, scrubbed, thinly sliced, soaked in warm water for 10 min
- ½ teaspoon garlic powder
- ½ teaspoon onion powder
- ½ teaspoon red chili powder
- ½ teaspoon curry powder
- 1 teaspoon of sea salt

- 1 tablespoon apple cider vinegar
- 2 tablespoons olive oil

Direction:

1. Drain the potato slices, pat dry, then place them in a large bowl, add remaining ingredients and toss until well coated.
2. Spread the potatoes in a single layer on a baking sheet and bake for 20 minutes until crispy, turning halfway.
3. Serve straight away.

Spinach and Artichoke Dip

Preparation time: 10 minutes

Cooking time: 25 minutes

Servings: 10

Nutritional Values (Per Serving):

- Calories:124 Cal
- Fat: 9 g
- Carbs: 8 g
- Protein: 5 g
- Fiber: 1 g

Ingredients:

- 28 ounces artichokes
- 1 small white onion, peeled, diced
- 1 1/2 cups cashews, soaked, drained
- 4 cups spinach
- 4 cloves of garlic, peeled
- 11 1/2 teaspoons salt
- 1/4 cup nutritional yeast

- 1 tablespoon olive oil
- 2 tablespoons lemon juice
- 1 1/2 cups coconut milk, unsweetened

Directions:

1. Cook onion and garlic in hot oil for 3 minutes until saute and then set aside until required.
2. Place cashews in a food processor; add 1 teaspoon salt, yeast, milk, and lemon juice and pulse until smooth.
3. Add spinach, onion mixture, and artichokes and pulse until the chunky mixture comes together.
4. Tip the dip in a heatproof dish and bake for 20 minutes at 425 degrees f until the top is browned and dip bubbles.
5. Serve straight away with vegetable sticks.

Chocolate-Covered Almonds

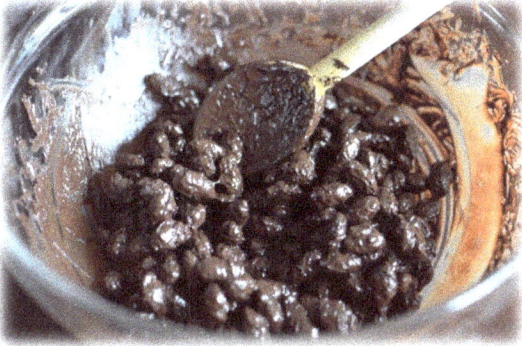

Preparation time: 1 hour and 45 minutes

Cooking time: 30 seconds

Servings: 4

Nutritional Values (Per Serving):

- Calories:286 Cal
- Fat: 22 g
- Carbs: 17 g
- Protein: 7 g
- Fiber: 5 g

Ingredients:

- 8 ounces almonds
- 1/2 teaspoon sea salt
- 6 ounces chocolate disks, semisweet, melted

Directions:

1. Microwave chocolate in a heatproof bowl for 30 seconds until it melts, then dip almonds in it, four at a time, and place them on a baking sheet.
2. Let almonds stand for 1 hour until hardened, then sprinkle with salt, and cool them in the refrigerator for 30 minutes.
3. Serve straight away.

Beans and Spinach Tacos

Preparation time: 10 minutes

Cooking time: 15 minutes

Servings: 4

Nutritional Values (Per Serving):

- Calories: 8 Cal
- Fat: 6 g
- Carbs: 34 g
- Protein: 9.9 g
- Fiber: 10 g

Ingredients:

- 12 ounces spinach
- 4 tablespoons cooked kidney beans
- ½ of medium red onion, peeled, chopped
- ½ teaspoon minced garlic
- 1 medium tomato, chopped
- 3 tablespoons chopped parsley
- ½ of avocado, sliced

- ½ teaspoon ground black pepper
- 1 teaspoon salt
- 2 tablespoons olive oil
- 4 slices of vegan brie cheese
- 4 tortillas, about 6-inches

Directions:

1. Take a skillet pan, place it over medium heat, add oil and when hot, add onion and cook for 10 minutes until softened.
2. Then stir in spinach, cook for 4 minutes until its leaf's wilts, then drain it and distribute evenly between tortillas.
3. Top evenly with remaining ingredients, season with black pepper and salt, drizzle with lemon juice and then serve.

Almond and Chia Pudding

Preparation time: 10 minutes

Cooking time: 15 minutes

Servings: 4

Nutritional Values (Per Serving):

- Calories 174
- Fat 12.1
- Fiber 3.2
- Carbs 3.9
- Protein 4.8

Ingredients:

- 1 tablespoon lime juice
- 1 tablespoon lime zest, grated
- 2 cups almond milk
- 2 tablespoons almonds, chopped

- 1 teaspoon almond extract
- ½ cup chia seeds
- 2 tablespoons stevia

Directions:

1. In a pan, mix the almond milk with the chia seeds, the almonds and the other ingredients, whisk, bring to a simmer and cook over medium heat for 15 minutes.
2. Divide the mix into bowls and serve cold.

Dates and Cocoa Bowls

Preparation time: 2 hours

Cooking time: 0 minutes

Servings: 6

Nutritional Values (Per Serving):

- Calories 141
- Fat 10.2
- Fiber 2.4
- Carbs 13.8
- Protein 1.4

Ingredients:

- 2 tablespoons avocado oil
- 1 cup coconut cream
- 1 teaspoon cocoa powder
- ½ cup dates, chopped
- 3 tablespoons stevia

Directions:

1. In a bowl, mix the cream with the oil, the cocoa, the cream and the other ingredients pulse well, divide into cups and keep in the fridge for 2 hours before serving.

Berries and Cherries Bowls

Preparation time: 10 minutes

Cooking time: 0 minutes

Servings: 4

Nutritional Values (Per Serving):

- Calories 122
- Fat 4
- Fiber 5.3
- Carbs 6.6
- Protein 4.5

Ingredients:

- 1 cup strawberries, halved
- 1 cup blackberries
- 1 cup cherries, pitted and halved
- ¼ cup coconut cream
- ¼ cup stevia
- 1 teaspoon vanilla extract

Directions:

1. In a bowl, combine the berries with the cherries and the other ingredients, toss, divide into smaller bowls and serve cold.

Cocoa Peach Cream

Preparation time: 10 minutes

Cooking time: 0 minutes

Servings: 4

Nutritional Values (Per Serving):

- Calories 172
- Fat 5.6
- Fiber 3.5
- Carbs 7.6
- Protein 4

Ingredients:

- 2 cups coconut cream
- 1/3 cup stevia
- ¾ cup cocoa powder
- Zest of 1 lime, grated
- 1 tablespoons lime juice
- 2 peaches, pitted and chopped

Directions:

1. In a blender, combine the cream with the stevia, the cocoa and the other ingredients, pulse well, divide into cups and serve cold.

Nuts and Seeds Pudding

Preparation time: 10 minutes

Cooking time: 20 minutes

Servings: 4

Nutritional Values (Per Serving):

- Calories 223
- Fat 8.1
- Fiber 3.4
- Carbs 7.6
- Protein 3.4

Ingredients:

- 2 cups cauliflower rice
- ¼ cup coconut cream
- 2 cups almond milk
- 1 teaspoon vanilla extract
- 3 tablespoons stevia
- ½ cup walnuts, chopped

- 1 tablespoon chia seeds
- Cooking spray

Directions:

1. In a pan, combine the cauliflower rice with the cream, the almond milk and the other ingredients, toss, bring to a simmer and cook over medium heat for 20 minutes.
2. Divide into bowls and serve cold.

Cashew Fudge

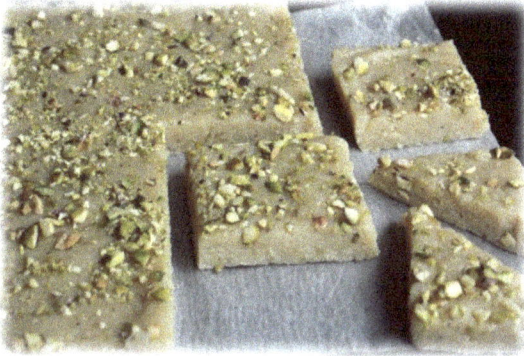

Preparation time: 3 hours

Cooking time: 0 minutes

Servings: 6

Nutritional Values (Per Serving):

- Calories 200
- Fat 4.5
- Fiber 3.4
- Carbs 13.5
- Protein 5

Ingredients:

- 1/3 cup cashew butter
- 1 cup coconut cream
- ½ cup cashews, soaked for 8 hours and drained
- 5 tablespoons lime juice
- ½ teaspoon lime zest, grated
- 1 tablespoons stevia

Directions:

1. In a bowl, mix the cashew butter with the cream, the cashews and the other ingredients and whisk well.
2. Line a muffin tray with parchment paper, scoop 1 tablespoon of the fudge mix in each of the muffin tins and freeze for 3 hours before serving.

Lime Berries Stew

Preparation time: 10 minutes

Cooking time: 20 minutes

Servings: 6

Nutritional Values (Per Serving):

- Calories 172
- Fat 7
- Fiber 3.4
- Carbs 8
- Protein 2.3

Ingredients:

- Zest of 1 lime, grated
- Juice of 1 lime
- 1 pint strawberries, halved
- 2 cups water
- 2 tablespoons stevia

Directions:

1. In a pan, combine the strawberries with the lime juice, the water and stevia, toss, bring to a simmer and cook over medium heat for 20 minutes.
2. Divide the stew into bowls and serve cold.

Apricots Cake

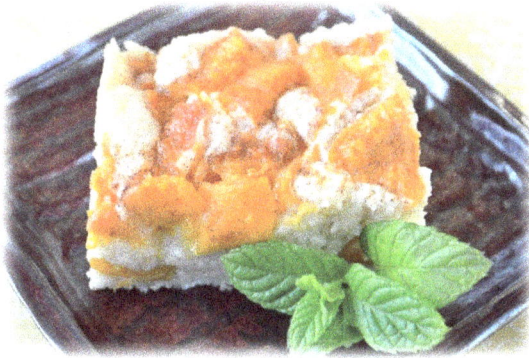

Preparation time: 10 minutes

Cooking time: 30 minutes

Servings: 8

Nutritional Values (Per Serving):

- Calories 221
- Fat 8.3
- Fiber 3.4
- Carbs 14.5
- Protein 5

Ingredients:

- ¾ cup stevia
- 2 cups coconut flour
- ¼ cup coconut oil, melted
- ½ cup almond milk
- 1 teaspoon baking powder
- 2 tablespoons flaxseed mixed with 3 tablespoons water
- ½ teaspoon vanilla extract
- Juice of 1 lime
- 2 cups apricots, chopped

Directions:

1. In a bowl, mix the flour with the coconut oil, the stevia and the other ingredients, whisk and pour into a cake pan lined with parchment paper.
2. Introduce in the oven at 375 degrees F, bake for 30 minutes, cool down, slice and serve.

Gorgonzola 'Blue' Cheese (vegan)

Preparation time: 24 hours

Cooking time: 20 minutes

Servings: 16

Nutritions:

- Calories: 101kcal
- Net Carbs: 2g
- Fat: 9.3g
- Protein: 2.3g
- Fiber: 1g
- Sugar: 0.9g

Ingredients:

- ½ cup macadamia nuts (unsalted)
- ½ cup pine nuts
- 1 cup raw cashews (unsalted)
- 1 capsule acidophilus (probiotic cheese culture)
- ½ tbsp. MCT oil
- ¼ cup unsweetened almond milk
- 1 tsp. ground black pepper
- 1 tsp. Himalayan salt
- 1 tsp. spirulina powder

Directions:

1. Cover the cashews with water in a small bowl and let sit for 4 to 6 hours. Rinse and drain the cashews after soaking. Make sure no water is left.
2. Preheat the oven to 350°F / 175°C, and line a baking sheet with parchment paper.
3. Spread the macadamia and pine nuts out on the baking sheet so they can roast evenly.
4. Put the baking sheet into the oven and roast the nuts for 8 minutes, until they are slightly browned.
5. Take the nuts out of the oven and allow them to cool down.
6. Grease a 3-inch cheese mold with the MCT oil and set it aside.

7. Add all ingredients—except the spirulina—to the blender or food processor. Blend on medium speed into a smooth mixture. Use a spatula to scrape down the sides of the blender to make sure all the **Ingredients:** get incorporated.

8. Transfer the cheese mixture into the greased cheese mold and sprinkle it with the spirulina powder. Use a small teaspoon to create blue marble veins on the cheese, and then cover the mold with parchment paper.

9. Place the cheese into a dehydrator and dehydrate the cheese at 90°F / 32°C for 24 hours.

10. Transfer the dehydrated cheese in the covered mold to the fridge. Allow the cheese to refrigerate for 12 hours.

11. Remove the cheese from the mold to serve in this condition, or, age the cheese in a wine cooler for up to 3 weeks. In case of aging the cheese, rub the outsides of the cheese with fresh sea salt. Refresh the salt every 2 days to prevent any mold. The cheese will develop a blue cheese-like taste, and by aging it, the cheese becomes even more delicious.

12. If the cheese is not aged, store it in airtight container and consume within 6

13. days.

14. Store the aged cheese in an airtight container and consume within 6 days, or for

15. a maximum of 60 days in the freezer and thaw at room temperature.

Zucchini & Ricotta Tart

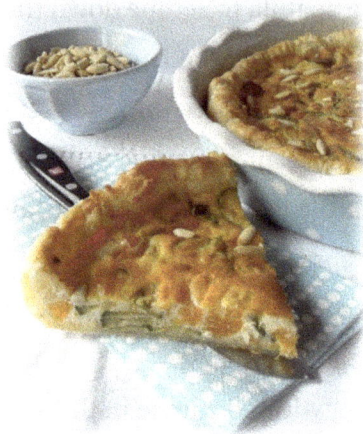

Preparation time: 25 minutes

Cooking time: about 1 hour

Servings: 8

Nutritions:

- Calories: 302
- Total Fats: 25.2g
- Carbohydrates: 7.9g
- Fiber: 3.1g
- Protein: 12.4g

Ingredients:

For the crust:

- 1¾ cups almond flour
- 1 tablespoon coconut flour
- ½ teaspoon garlic powder
- ¼ teaspoon salt
- ¼ cup melted butter

For the filling:

- 1 medium-large zucchini, thinly sliced cross-wise (use a mandolin if you have one)
- ½ teaspoon salt
- 8 ounces ricotta
- 3 large eggs
- ¼ cup whipping cream
- 2 cloves garlic, minced
- 1 teaspoon fresh dill, minced
- Additional salt and pepper to taste
- ½ cup shredded parmesan

Directions:

For the crust:

1. Preheat oven to 325°F.
2. Lightly spray 9-inch ceramic or glass tart pan with cooking spray.
3. Combine the almond flour, coconut flour, garlic powder and salt in a large bowl.
4. Add the butter and stir until dough resembles coarse crumbs.
5. Press the dough gently into the tart pan, trimming away any excess.
6. Bake 15 minutes then remove from the oven and let cool.

To make the filling:

7. While crust is baking, put the zucchini slices into a colander and sprinkle each layer with a little salt. Let sit and drain for 30 minutes.
8. Place salted zucchini between double layers of paper towels and gently press down to remove any excess water.
9. Place the ricotta, eggs, whipping cream, garlic, dill, salt and pepper in a bowl and stir well to combine. Add almost all the zucchini slices, reserving about 25-30 for layering on top.
10. Transfer mixture into cooled crust. Top with the remaining zucchini slices, slightly overlapping.
11. Sprinkle with parmesan cheese.
12. Bake 60 to 70 minutes or until center is no longer wobbly and a toothpick comes out clean.
13. Cut into slices and serve.

Eggplant Noodles with Sesame Tofu

Preparation time: 25 minutes

Cooking time: 20-22 minutes

Servings: 4

Nutritions:

- Calories: 293
- Total Fats: 24.4g
- Carbohydrates: 12.2g
- Fiber: 5.3g
- Protein: 11g

Ingredients:

- 1 pound block firm tofu
- 1 cup chopped cilantro
- 3 tablespoons rice vinegar
- 4 tablespoons toasted sesame oil
- 2 cloves garlic, finely minced

- 1 teaspoon crushed red pepper flakes
- 2 teaspoons Swerve confectioners
- 1 whole eggplant
- 1 tablespoon olive oil
- Salt and pepper to taste
- ¼ cup sesame seeds
- ¼ cup soy sauce

Directions:

1. Preheat oven to 200°F.
2. Remove the block of tofu from packaging. Wrap the tofu in a kitchen towel or paper towels and place a heavy object on top, like a pan or canned goods (alternatively, you can use a tofu press). Let the tofu drain for at least 15 minutes.
3. In a large mixing bowl, add about ¼ cup of cilantro, 3 tablespoons rice vinegar, 2 tablespoons toasted sesame oil, minced garlic, crushed red pepper flakes, and Swerve; whisk together.
4. Peel and julienne the eggplant. You can julienne roughly by hand, or you can use a mandolin with a julienne attachment to cut the eggplant into thin noodles.
5. Add the eggplant into bowl with marinade; toss to coat.
6. Place a skillet over medium-low heat and add olive oil. Once the oil is heated, add the eggplant and cook until it softens. The eggplant will soak up all the liquids, so if you have issues

with it sticking to the pan, feel free to add a little more sesame or olive oil. Just be sure to adjust your nutrition tracking.

7. Turn the oven off. Add the remaining cilantro into the eggplant then place the noodles in an oven safe dish. Cover with a lid or foil and place into the oven to keep warm.

8. Pour off fat from skillet then wipe skillet clean with paper towels. Place it back on the stovetop to heat up again.

9. Unwrap the tofu then cut into 8 slices. Spread sesame seeds over a large plate. Press both sides of each tofu slice into the sesame seeds to coat evenly. Transfer to a plate.

10. Pour 2 tablespoons of sesame oil into the skillet.

11. Arrange the tofu slices in a single layer in the skillet and cook on medium-low for about 5 minutes or until they start to crisp. With a spatula, carefully turn them over and cook for about 5 minutes on the other side.

12. Pour ¼ cup of soy sauce into the pan and coat the pieces of tofu. Cook until the tofu slices look browned and caramelized with the soy sauce.

13. To serve, remove the eggplant noodles from the oven, divide them among plates and place the tofu on top.

Cheesy Crustless Quiche

Preparation time: 30 minutes

Cooking time: 1 hour

Servings: 6

Nutritions:

- Calories: 301
- Total Fats: 20g
- Carbohydrates: 8g
- Fiber: 1g
- Protein: 23g
- Sugar: 4g

Ingredients:

- 6 small Roma tomatoes
- ½ cup thinly sliced green onion
- 6 large eggs, beaten
- ¼ teaspoon Italian Herb Blend
- ½ teaspoon Spike Seasoning (optional but recommended)
- ½ cup half and half

- 1 cup cottage cheese
- 2 cups shredded Swiss cheese
- ¼ cup finely grated Parmesan cheese
- ¼ cup thinly sliced basil
- Salt and fresh-ground black pepper to taste

Directions:

1. Preheat oven to 350°F. Coat a 9-10″ glass or crockery pie dish with non-stick spray.
2. Cut 3 small Roma tomatoes in half lengthwise and scoop out the seeds. Pat the interior dry with paper towels and then chop the tomatoes.
3. Break the eggs into a large bowl, add the half and half, Italian Herb Blend, Spike Seasonings, salt and pepper. Whisk until combined.
4. Stir in the cottage cheese, Swiss cheese, Parmesan cheese, chopped tomatoes, and green onion.
5. Pour into the prepared pie dish and bake for 30 minutes.
6. Meanwhile, thinly slice 3 remaining small Roma tomatoes and put on a plate between layers of paper towel. Gently press to help draw out the moisture.
7. After 30 minutes, remove the quiche from the oven and distribute sliced tomatoes and sliced basil on top of the quiche.

8. Return to oven and bake an additional 30 minutes or slightly more if the center doesn't seem set enough.
9. Turn oven to Broil and cook for a minute or two until browned. But keep a close eye on it so the basil does not burn.
10. Allow the quiche to sit for 5-10 minutes before cutting.
11. Serve warm or at room temperature.

Rutabaga Hash Browns

Preparation time: 20 minutes

Cooking time: 10 minutes

Servings: 6

Nutritions:

- Calories: 114
- Total Fats: 8g
- Carbohydrates: 7g
- Fiber: 2g
- Protein: 3g

Ingredients:

- 1 large rutabaga (about 1 pound)
- ¼ cup finely grated Parmesan cheese
- 1½ teaspoons dried minced onion
- ½ teaspoon sea salt
- ¼ teaspoon black pepper
- 3 tablespoons avocado oil (or your preferred high-heat tolerant oil)

Directions:

1. Peel the outer skin from the rutabaga. Chop into about 8 equal pieces.
2. Bring a medium pot of salted water to a boil. Add peeled & chopped rutabaga and cook over medium- high heat for 10 minutes.
3. Place the rutabaga pieces in a colander or strainer and rinse them under cold running water then pat dry with a few paper towels.
4. Shred the rutabaga with either a grater or a food processor equipped with a shredding blade.
5. Add Parmesan cheese and minced onion to shredded rutabaga, season with salt and pepper, and mix to combine.
6. Place a large frying pan over medium-low heat and add about 1 tablespoon of oil. Once the oil is heated, add shredded rutabaga, and cook, working in batches, until crisp and golden brown on one side, 3 to 4 minutes. If desired, gently press the layer down with a spatula. Then use a spatula to flip the rutabaga. Continue to cook until they are golden brown on the bottom, about 3 minutes.
7. Serve immediately.

Twice Baked Spaghetti Squash

Preparation time: 15 minutes

Cooking time: 55 minutes

Servings: 6

Nutritions:

- Calories: 173
- Total Fats: 12g
- Carbohydrates: 10g
- Fiber: 2g

Ingredients:

- 2 pounds spaghetti squash
- 1 tablespoon olive oil
- ¾ cup pecorino romano cheese, shredded (or parmesan)
- 1 cup mozzarella cheese, shredded
- 1 teaspoon onion powder
- 1 tablespoon butter
- 2 tablespoons fresh thyme leaves
- 3 cloves garlic, minced

- ½ teaspoon salt
- ¼ teaspoon pepper

Directions:

1. Preheat oven to 400°F.
2. Use a fork to poke a few holes around the spaghetti squash. Put in the microwave and cook for a minute to soften a bit.
3. On a cutting board, cut off the end of squash, then cut in half lengthwise. Use a spoon to scrape the pulp and seeds. Rub inside surface with olive oil.
4. Place each piece of squash, cut side down, onto the baking sheet.
5. Bake 40-50 minutes or until it has become fork tender.
6. Let cool for a bit and then use a fork to remove all the strands of spaghetti squash into a mixing bowl.
7. Put pecorino romano cheese and mozzarella cheese into small dish then add HALF the cheese mixture to the bowl with squash. Add butter, minced garlic, onion powder, fresh thyme, salt and pepper. Using a fork, mash and mix thoroughly to combine everything with the squash flesh.
8. Spoon this squash mixture back into the skins on a baking sheet pan.
9. Sprinkle tops with the rest of the cheese mixture and return to oven. Broil 5-6 minutes or until the cheese is melted and starting to brown.
10. Serve hot.

www.ingramcontent.com/pod-product-compliance
Lightning Source LLC
Chambersburg PA
CBHW050746030426
42336CB00012B/1682